Copyright © 2023 by Herman Strange (Author)

All rights reserved. This book or any portion thereof may not be reproduced or used in any manner whatsoever without the express written permission of the publisher except for the use of brief quotations in a book review.

This book is copyright protected. This is only for personal use. You cannot amend, distributor, sell, use, quote or paraphrase any part or the content within this book without the consent of the author. Please note the information contained within this document is for educational and entertainment purposes only. Every attempt has been made to provide accurate, up to date and reliable complete information. No warranties of any kind are expressed or implied.

Readers acknowledge that the author is not engaging in the rendering of legal, financial, medical or professional advice. The content of this book has been derived from various sources. Please consult a licensed professional before attempting any techniques outlined in this book.

By reading this document, the readers agree that under no circumstances are the author responsible for any losses, direct or indirect, which are incurred as a result of the use of information contained within this document, including but not limited to errors, omissions or inaccuracies.

Thank you very much for reading this book.

Title: *Moving for Health-Effective Ways to Incorporate Physical Activity into Your Daily Routine*

Subtitle: *Strategies for Staying Active in Today's World*

Series: Healthy Habits for Life: Building Sustainable Habits for Optimal Health and Wellness

Author: Serenity Tanner

Table of Contents

Introduction 5
   Importance of Physical Activity 6
   Purpose of the Book 8
   Overview of Comparison Methods 10

Chapter 1: Fitness Trackers 11
   How They Work and What They Track 11
   Pros and Cons 13
   Popular Brands 15

Chapter 2: Exercise Apps 17
   How They Work and What They Offer 17
   Pros and Cons 19
   Popular Apps 21

Chapter 3: Smart Home Gym Equipment 24
   How It Works and What It Offers 24
   Pros and Cons 26
   Popular Equipment 29

Chapter 4: Virtual Fitness Classes 34
   How They Work and What They Offer 34
   Pros and Cons 37
   Popular Classes 40

Chapter 5: Pedometers 43
   How They Work and What They Track 43
   Pros and Cons 45

Popular Pedometers *48*

Chapter 6: Exercise Video Games **50**

How They Work and What They Offer *50*

Pros and Cons *53*

Popular Games *56*

Chapter 7: Smart Watches **58**

How They Work and What They Track *58*

Pros and Cons *60*

Popular Watches *62*

Chapter 8: Comparing and Contrasting Methods .. **68**

Summary of Pros and Cons *68*

Criteria for Comparison *75*

Recommendations for Different Needs *77*

Conclusion **79**

Recap of Importance of Physical Activity *79*

Final Thoughts and Recommendations *81*

Potential References **83**

Introduction

Staying active is one of the most important things you can do for your health. In a world where we spend most of our time sitting and looking at screens, it can be hard to prioritize physical activity. However, incorporating exercise and movement into your daily routine can have a significant impact on your physical and mental well-being. In this chapter, we'll explore the benefits of physical activity and why it should be a priority in your life.

Importance of Physical Activity

Physical activity is essential for maintaining a healthy body and mind. Regular exercise can help prevent chronic diseases such as heart disease, diabetes, and obesity. It can also improve your mood, reduce stress, and increase your energy levels. Here are some of the key benefits of physical activity:

Reduces the risk of chronic disease: Physical activity can help prevent chronic diseases such as heart disease, stroke, diabetes, and cancer. Regular exercise helps to maintain healthy blood pressure, cholesterol levels, and blood sugar levels, which can reduce the risk of developing these diseases.

Helps manage weight: Physical activity can help you maintain a healthy weight or lose weight if needed. Exercise helps to burn calories, build muscle, and increase metabolism, which can all contribute to weight loss.

Improves mental health: Exercise has been shown to reduce symptoms of anxiety and depression, as well as improve overall mood. Physical activity also releases endorphins, which are the body's natural feel-good chemicals.

Increases energy levels: Regular exercise can increase energy levels and reduce fatigue. Exercise helps to improve circulation, which can deliver more oxygen and nutrients to your body's tissues, leading to increased energy levels.

Improves sleep: Exercise can help you fall asleep faster and stay asleep longer. Physical activity can also improve the quality of your sleep, leading to increased alertness and productivity during the day.

These are just a few of the many benefits of physical activity. Incorporating regular exercise into your daily routine can have a significant impact on your overall health and well-being. In the following chapters, we'll explore different methods for staying active and building a sustainable exercise routine that works for you.

Purpose of the Book

The purpose of this book is to provide readers with a comprehensive guide to incorporating physical activity into their daily routines. In today's world, it can be difficult to find the time and motivation to stay active, but the benefits of doing so are numerous. Regular physical activity has been shown to improve overall health, reduce the risk of chronic diseases, and even improve mental health.

Unfortunately, many people are unsure of where to start when it comes to incorporating physical activity into their lives. There are countless options available, from fitness trackers and exercise apps to smart home gym equipment and virtual fitness classes. This book aims to provide a detailed comparison of these methods, along with their pros and cons, to help readers choose the best option for their needs.

The purpose of this book is not to promote one method over another, but rather to provide a comprehensive overview of the options available so that readers can make an informed decision. Different people have different needs, preferences, and lifestyles, and what works for one person may not work for another. By providing a detailed comparison of the various methods, readers can identify which ones are most likely to work for them.

Another goal of this book is to provide readers with the knowledge and tools they need to build sustainable habits for optimal health and wellness. Incorporating physical activity into your daily routine is not a one-time event, but a habit that needs to be cultivated over time. By providing readers with the information and resources they need to build sustainable habits, this book can help readers achieve long-term success in their fitness journeys.

Overall, the purpose of this book is to empower readers to take control of their physical health by providing them with the information and resources they need to incorporate physical activity into their daily routines. Whether you're a fitness enthusiast or a beginner, this book can help you find the method that works best for your needs and achieve your fitness goals.

Overview of Comparison Methods

In this book, we will explore various methods for incorporating physical activity into your daily routine, including fitness trackers, exercise apps, smart home gym equipment, virtual fitness classes, pedometers, exercise video games, and smartwatches.

With the proliferation of technology and the growing demand for convenience, there has been a surge in the number of devices and tools designed to help people stay active and healthy. This abundance of options can be overwhelming, and it can be difficult to know which methods are most effective for your specific needs.

To help you navigate this landscape, we will provide an overview of each of the comparison methods in this book, including how they work, what they offer, their pros and cons, and their popularity. We will also compare and contrast these methods based on specific criteria, and provide recommendations for different needs and preferences.

By the end of this book, you will have a clear understanding of the various methods for staying active in today's world and will be able to choose the ones that work best for you.

Chapter 1: Fitness Trackers
How They Work and What They Track

Fitness trackers have become increasingly popular in recent years, with many people turning to these devices as a way to monitor and track their physical activity. But how exactly do fitness trackers work, and what kind of data do they track?

At their core, fitness trackers are wearable devices that use sensors to track various metrics related to physical activity. These sensors can include accelerometers, gyroscopes, and heart rate monitors, among others. The data collected by these sensors is then processed and analyzed by the device's software, which provides the user with feedback on their activity levels.

One of the primary metrics that fitness trackers track is steps taken. This is accomplished through the use of an accelerometer, which measures the movement of the user's body as they walk or run. Based on the number of steps detected, the device can provide an estimate of the user's daily activity level.

Many fitness trackers also track distance traveled, which is calculated based on the user's stride length and the number of steps taken. This metric can be useful for individuals who are looking to increase their overall activity levels and set distance-based goals.

In addition to steps and distance, fitness trackers can also track the user's heart rate. This is typically accomplished using a combination of optical sensors and algorithms that analyze changes in blood flow beneath the skin. Heart rate monitoring can be useful for individuals who are looking to track their fitness levels and ensure that they are getting enough cardiovascular exercise.

Some fitness trackers also track sleep patterns, which can be useful for individuals who are looking to improve their overall health and well-being. These devices use a combination of sensors to detect the user's movement and heart rate during sleep, which can provide insights into the quality and duration of their sleep.

Overall, fitness trackers are powerful tools for individuals looking to improve their physical activity levels and overall health. By tracking metrics such as steps, distance, heart rate, and sleep patterns, these devices can help users gain a better understanding of their activity levels and make informed decisions about their health and wellness.

Pros and Cons

Pros:

Accountability: Fitness trackers provide a way to track progress and hold oneself accountable to fitness goals. This can provide motivation to stay on track and work towards achieving fitness objectives.

Goal setting: Many fitness trackers allow users to set personalized fitness goals, which can help guide workout routines and focus on achieving specific milestones. Setting and achieving goals can help with motivation and provide a sense of accomplishment.

Activity tracking: Fitness trackers can monitor daily activity, including steps taken, distance traveled, and calories burned. This can provide insight into overall physical activity levels and help identify areas for improvement.

Heart rate monitoring: Some fitness trackers include heart rate monitors, which can provide valuable information during workouts, such as tracking heart rate zones and monitoring intensity levels.

Sleep tracking: Many fitness trackers also have the ability to track sleep patterns, including duration and quality of sleep. This information can help users identify patterns and adjust habits to improve sleep quality.

Cons:

Inaccuracy: Some fitness trackers can be inaccurate, leading to false data or inaccurate readings. This can be frustrating and may lead to incorrect goal setting or poor performance tracking.

Cost: Fitness trackers can be expensive, and the cost may not be justified for some users who do not require the added features or benefits.

Battery life: Some fitness trackers require frequent charging or have short battery life, which can be inconvenient and disrupt the tracking process.

Comfort: Depending on the design and fit of the fitness tracker, it may be uncomfortable to wear for extended periods of time, especially during workouts.

Data overload: With so much data being collected and displayed, it can be overwhelming and difficult to make sense of the information. This may lead to confusion and frustration, rather than providing useful insights.

Overall, fitness trackers can be a valuable tool for tracking fitness progress, setting and achieving goals, and monitoring overall physical activity. However, it's important to weigh the pros and cons before investing in a fitness tracker, and to choose one that best meets individual needs and preferences.

Popular Brands

When it comes to fitness trackers, there are many brands to choose from. Each brand has its own unique features and benefits, and the best one for you will depend on your individual needs and preferences. Here are some of the most popular fitness tracker brands on the market today:

Fitbit: Fitbit is one of the most well-known fitness tracker brands, and for good reason. Their devices offer a wide range of features, including step tracking, heart rate monitoring, and sleep tracking. Fitbit also has a large community of users, which can be helpful for those who want to connect with others and share their fitness journey.

Garmin: Garmin is another popular brand that offers a range of fitness trackers. Their devices are known for their accuracy and durability, making them a great choice for those who want a reliable tracker that can withstand tough workouts. Garmin's devices also offer advanced features, such as GPS tracking and personalized coaching.

Apple: While not exclusively a fitness tracker brand, Apple's smartwatches offer a range of fitness tracking features, including heart rate monitoring, step tracking, and workout tracking. Apple's watches also offer a range of other features, such as mobile payments and access to apps, making them a versatile choice for those who want a multifunctional device.

Samsung: Samsung's fitness trackers offer a range of features, including heart rate monitoring, sleep tracking, and step tracking. They also have a sleek and stylish design, making them a good choice for those who want a tracker that looks good both in and out of the gym.

Xiaomi: Xiaomi is a Chinese brand that has gained popularity in recent years for their affordable fitness trackers. Despite their low price point, Xiaomi's trackers offer a range of features, including step tracking and heart rate monitoring. They may not have all the advanced features of more expensive brands, but they are a good choice for those who want a basic tracker without breaking the bank.

Other popular fitness tracker brands include Polar, Withings, and Misfit. When choosing a fitness tracker, it's important to consider your budget, the features you need, and the style and design of the device. With so many options to choose from, there is sure to be a fitness tracker that meets your needs and helps you achieve your fitness goals.

Chapter 2: Exercise Apps
How They Work and What They Offer

Exercise apps are becoming increasingly popular as people seek more convenient and flexible ways to stay active. They are essentially mobile applications that help users track their exercise routines, set goals, and monitor progress. These apps work on a wide range of devices, including smartphones, tablets, and wearable technology like smartwatches.

There are a variety of features that exercise apps offer, and they can be tailored to suit different needs and preferences. Some of the most common features include:

Customized Workouts: Many exercise apps allow users to customize their workouts by selecting the type of exercise, duration, and intensity level.

Goal Setting: Users can set goals for themselves, such as a desired weight loss or number of steps per day, and track their progress.

Social Sharing: Some exercise apps allow users to share their progress with friends and family on social media or within the app's community.

Virtual Coaching: Some apps offer virtual coaching or personalized training plans based on a user's goals and fitness level.

Integration with Other Apps and Devices: Many exercise apps can be integrated with other health and fitness apps, as well as wearable technology like fitness trackers and smartwatches.

Gamification: Some apps use gamification features, such as challenges and rewards, to motivate users to stay active and reach their goals.

Overall, exercise apps are a convenient and accessible way to stay active and monitor progress towards fitness goals. They offer a wide range of features that can be customized to suit individual needs, and can be used in combination with other health and fitness apps and devices. However, like all technology, there are some potential downsides to consider as well.

Pros and Cons

Pros:

Convenience: One of the biggest advantages of exercise apps is that they can be used at any time and from anywhere. This means that users can work out at home or on-the-go, without having to go to a gym or fitness center.

Personalization: Exercise apps offer a wide range of workout routines and plans that can be customized to meet the specific needs and goals of each user. This means that users can tailor their workouts to focus on certain areas of the body, or to achieve a specific fitness goal.

Cost-effective: Most exercise apps are either free or cost significantly less than a gym membership or personal trainer. This makes them a more cost-effective option for those who are on a budget.

Motivation: Many exercise apps have features that help users stay motivated, such as progress tracking, reminders, and virtual rewards. This can help users stay committed to their fitness goals and stick to their workout routines.

Cons:

Limited interaction: While exercise apps can offer personalized workout plans, they lack the personalized attention and interaction that a personal trainer can provide.

This means that users may not receive feedback on their form or technique, which could increase their risk of injury.

Lack of variety: Some exercise apps may not offer a wide variety of workouts or routines, which could lead to boredom and a lack of motivation to continue using the app.

Technical issues: Like all technology, exercise apps may experience technical difficulties, such as crashing or glitches. This can be frustrating for users who are in the middle of a workout.

Reliance on technology: Exercise apps require a reliable internet connection and a functional device. If either of these are not available, users may not be able to access their workout plans.

Overall, exercise apps can be a great option for those looking for a cost-effective and convenient way to incorporate physical activity into their daily routine. However, it is important to weigh the pros and cons before deciding if an exercise app is the right choice for your fitness goals and lifestyle.

Popular Apps

When it comes to exercise apps, there are countless options available, each with their own unique features and benefits. Here are some of the most popular exercise apps that you might want to consider:

Nike Training Club: The Nike Training Club app offers a wide range of workouts, including strength training, yoga, and cardio, that can be customized to your fitness level and goals. The app also provides personalized recommendations based on your workout history and preferences.

Peloton: While Peloton is best known for its high-end exercise equipment, the company also offers an app that provides access to a wide range of live and on-demand workouts, including cycling, running, strength training, and yoga. The app also includes features like progress tracking and personalized coaching.

MyFitnessPal: MyFitnessPal is a comprehensive fitness app that allows you to track your workouts, monitor your nutrition, and set and track your fitness goals. The app also includes a large database of foods and exercises, making it easy to log your meals and workouts.

Fitbod: Fitbod is a weightlifting app that creates customized workout plans based on your goals, fitness level, and available equipment. The app also tracks your progress and adjusts your workouts over time to help you reach your goals.

Strava: Strava is a social fitness app that allows you to track your workouts, connect with friends, and join challenges and groups. The app also provides insights and analytics on your workouts, as well as personalized training plans.

Daily Burn: Daily Burn is a workout app that offers a wide range of live and on-demand workouts, including dance, yoga, and strength training. The app also includes features like progress tracking, personalized coaching, and a community of users for support and motivation.

Sworkit: Sworkit is a workout app that provides customizable workouts based on your fitness level and goals. The app also includes features like progress tracking, personalized coaching, and the ability to create your own custom workouts.

Aaptiv: Aaptiv is a workout app that offers audio-based fitness classes, including running, cycling, and strength training. The app also includes personalized coaching, progress tracking, and a large library of workouts to choose from.

Zombies, Run!: Zombies, Run! is a unique app that combines fitness with storytelling. The app turns your workouts into a mission to survive a zombie apocalypse, with audio cues and instructions that guide you through the story and your workout.

Seven: Seven is a workout app that provides short, seven-minute workouts that can be done anywhere, anytime. The app also includes personalized coaching, progress tracking, and a large library of workouts to choose from.

These are just a few of the most popular exercise apps available, but there are many others to choose from. When deciding on an app, consider your fitness goals, preferences, and available equipment, as well as the app's features and user reviews.

Chapter 3: Smart Home Gym Equipment
How It Works and What It Offers

Smart home gym equipment is an increasingly popular option for those looking to incorporate physical activity into their daily routine. This equipment is designed to offer a convenient, at-home workout experience that can be tailored to the user's individual needs and preferences.

One of the key features of smart home gym equipment is its ability to provide customized workouts. With the help of technology, these machines can adjust their settings based on the user's fitness level, goals, and preferences. This means that individuals can receive a workout that is tailored to their specific needs, whether that be a cardio-focused routine or a strength-training session.

Another benefit of smart home gym equipment is its convenience. With a machine in the comfort of one's own home, individuals can avoid the hassle and expense of going to a gym. This can be particularly beneficial for those with busy schedules or limited access to transportation.

Smart home gym equipment often comes with a variety of features and functions designed to enhance the workout experience. For example, some machines may offer built-in screens that allow users to access virtual classes or workouts, while others may include features such as heart rate monitoring, adjustable resistance levels, and personalized coaching.

Some types of smart home gym equipment may also include interactive features that allow users to compete with friends, track progress, and earn rewards for hitting certain milestones. This can provide an added layer of motivation and accountability to the workout experience.

Overall, smart home gym equipment offers a convenient and customizable way for individuals to incorporate physical activity into their daily routine. With its variety of features and functions, this equipment can provide a personalized workout experience that is both effective and enjoyable.

Pros and Cons

Smart home gym equipment has gained significant popularity in recent years, thanks to advancements in technology that have made it possible to create equipment that is compact, versatile, and easy to use. However, just like any other fitness equipment, there are both pros and cons to using smart home gym equipment. In this section, we will explore some of the advantages and disadvantages of using this type of equipment.

Pros:

Convenience: Smart home gym equipment allows you to work out in the comfort of your own home, at any time of the day or night. This can be particularly beneficial for people who have busy schedules or live in areas with inclement weather.

Customization: Many smart home gym equipment models come with a variety of settings and programs that can be customized to fit your specific fitness goals. This allows you to create a workout plan that is tailored to your unique needs and preferences.

Variety: Smart home gym equipment comes in a variety of forms, from treadmills and stationary bikes to rowing machines and ellipticals. This means that you can choose the equipment that best suits your interests and fitness level.

Space-saving: Unlike traditional gym equipment, smart home gym equipment is designed to be compact and easily stored when not in use. This makes it a great option for people who don't have a lot of space in their homes.

Cons:

Cost: Smart home gym equipment can be more expensive than traditional gym equipment. The added features and technology can drive up the price, making it unaffordable for some.

Maintenance: Just like any other fitness equipment, smart home gym equipment requires regular maintenance to keep it in good working condition. This can be time-consuming and costly, especially if you're not familiar with the maintenance requirements.

Limited instruction: Smart home gym equipment often comes with limited instruction or guidance on how to use it properly. This can be a problem for beginners who are not familiar with how to operate the equipment.

Limited interaction: Smart home gym equipment lacks the social aspect of traditional gyms, where people can interact and motivate each other to work harder. This can make it difficult to stay motivated and committed to your fitness goals.

Despite these cons, smart home gym equipment remains a popular option for many people who want to work out at home. By weighing the pros and cons, you can determine whether this type of equipment is right for you and your fitness goals.

Popular Equipment

Smart home gym equipment has become increasingly popular in recent years, with more and more people choosing to work out at home instead of going to a gym. There are a variety of different types of equipment available, ranging from cardio machines to strength training equipment. In this section, we will discuss some of the most popular types of smart home gym equipment.

Treadmills

Treadmills are one of the most popular types of home gym equipment, and for good reason. They allow you to get a great cardio workout without having to leave your home. Many treadmills come equipped with various features, such as heart rate monitors and pre-programmed workouts, making it easy to customize your workout to your specific fitness goals.

One of the downsides of treadmills, however, is that they can be quite expensive. In addition, they take up a lot of space and can be difficult to move once they are set up.

Ellipticals

Ellipticals are another popular type of cardio machine that can provide a low-impact workout for those who want to avoid putting too much stress on their joints. They work by simulating a running motion, but without the impact of your feet hitting the ground.

Like treadmills, many ellipticals come with pre-programmed workouts and heart rate monitors, and some models can even be connected to the internet to download new workouts and track your progress.

One of the main downsides of ellipticals is that they can be quite expensive. In addition, they can take up a lot of space and may be difficult to move once they are set up.

Stationary Bikes

Stationary bikes are another popular type of cardio machine that are commonly found in home gyms. They offer a low-impact workout that can be customized to your fitness level, and many come with features such as adjustable resistance levels and pre-programmed workouts.

One of the main benefits of stationary bikes is that they are relatively compact and easy to move around. They are also generally less expensive than treadmills and ellipticals.

One potential downside of stationary bikes is that they can be uncomfortable to sit on for extended periods of time. It is important to choose a model with a comfortable seat and handlebars to avoid discomfort during your workout.

Strength Training Equipment

In addition to cardio machines, there are also a variety of smart home gym equipment options for strength training. These can include everything from dumbbells and resistance bands to larger, more complex machines such as multi-gyms and cable machines.

The main benefit of strength training equipment is that it allows you to target specific muscle groups and build strength and muscle mass. Many machines also come with built-in safety features to prevent injury.

One downside of strength training equipment is that it can be quite expensive, especially if you are looking for a machine that targets multiple muscle groups. In addition, many machines can be quite large and take up a lot of space in your home gym.

Multi-Purpose Machines

For those who want a full-body workout without having to purchase multiple machines, multi-purpose machines are a popular option. These machines typically offer a variety of different exercises, including cardio and strength training, all in one piece of equipment.

One of the main benefits of multi-purpose machines is that they can save space in your home gym. They also offer a comprehensive workout that can target multiple muscle groups.

One potential downside of multi-purpose machines is that they can be quite expensive, and may not offer the same level of customization as individual machines for specific exercises.

Overall, there are several smart home gym equipment options available on the market. Here are some of the most popular:

Peloton Bike: Peloton is a popular brand that offers high-quality, interactive home gym equipment. Their signature product is the Peloton bike, which has a large screen that allows you to participate in live and on-demand classes.

Mirror: Mirror is a smart gym that provides a sleek, full-length mirror that doubles as an interactive workout device. It comes with a monthly subscription service that offers live and on-demand classes.

Tonal: Tonal is a digital strength training machine that uses digital weights and adjustable arms to provide a customizable workout experience. It also has an AI coach that adapts to your fitness level and goals.

NordicTrack Commercial Series: NordicTrack is a well-known brand in the fitness industry that offers a range of home gym equipment. Their commercial series includes treadmills, ellipticals, and bikes that come with large touchscreens and iFit subscription services.

Bowflex Max Trainer: The Bowflex Max Trainer is a compact elliptical machine that provides a high-intensity, low-impact workout. It also comes with a subscription service that offers customized workouts and coaching.

These are just a few examples of the popular smart home gym equipment options available. Each has its pros and cons, and the best choice depends on individual preferences and needs.

Chapter 4: Virtual Fitness Classes
How They Work and What They Offer

Virtual fitness classes are becoming increasingly popular for individuals who prefer to exercise at home, on their own schedule, and with the guidance of a professional trainer. These classes are designed to be engaging and effective, with a wide range of workouts and styles to suit different fitness levels and preferences. In this chapter, we'll explore how virtual fitness classes work, and what they have to offer for those seeking a convenient and effective way to stay fit.

Virtual fitness classes are essentially live or recorded workout sessions that are broadcast online for participants to follow along at home. These classes are often led by professional trainers or fitness instructors who guide participants through a specific workout routine. Many virtual fitness classes can be accessed through online platforms or fitness apps, and can be performed with minimal equipment. Some popular virtual fitness class options include yoga, high-intensity interval training (HIIT), dance fitness, strength training, and even guided meditation.

One of the key benefits of virtual fitness classes is the flexibility they offer. Participants can join a class at any time that suits them, and don't need to worry about traveling to a gym or studio. This is particularly beneficial for people with busy schedules, those with limited access to fitness facilities, or those who prefer to exercise in the comfort of their own home. Additionally, virtual fitness classes typically require minimal equipment, making them a cost-effective option for those who may not want to invest in expensive fitness equipment or gym memberships.

Another advantage of virtual fitness classes is the ability to choose from a wide range of workout styles and formats. With options ranging from yoga and pilates to high-intensity interval training and dance fitness, individuals can find a workout that suits their fitness level and personal preferences. Virtual fitness classes also often incorporate music and other motivational tools to keep participants engaged and motivated throughout the session.

In addition to being convenient and engaging, virtual fitness classes can also be a great way to stay accountable to a fitness routine. Many classes are designed to be interactive, with opportunities for participants to ask questions and receive feedback from the instructor. This can be particularly helpful for those who may struggle with self-motivation or need additional guidance to stay on track with their fitness goals.

Overall, virtual fitness classes offer a convenient and effective way to stay active and engaged with a fitness routine. With a wide range of workout options and the ability to join classes at any time, individuals can find a workout that suits their preferences and schedule. Whether you're looking to try a new workout style, need extra motivation to stay active, or simply prefer the convenience of at-home workouts, virtual fitness classes are a great option to consider.

Pros and Cons

Pros:

Convenience: One of the biggest advantages of virtual fitness classes is convenience. Users can attend classes from the comfort of their own homes, without having to worry about travel time or distance.

Flexibility: Virtual fitness classes are available on demand, making them a flexible option for people with busy schedules. Users can choose from a variety of classes and times that fit their needs.

Variety: Virtual fitness classes offer a wide range of classes to choose from, including yoga, dance, HIIT, and more. This allows users to switch up their workout routine and find a class that they enjoy.

Access: Virtual fitness classes are accessible to people of all fitness levels, making them an inclusive option for those who may not feel comfortable attending an in-person class.

Cost-effective: Virtual fitness classes are often more cost-effective than in-person classes, as users do not have to pay for a gym membership or travel expenses.

Cons:

Technical issues: Virtual fitness classes require a stable internet connection, and technical issues can arise during the class, which can interrupt the workout.

Limited social interaction: Virtual fitness classes do not provide the same level of social interaction that in-person classes do. Users may feel isolated and miss the social aspect of working out in a group.

Lack of personalized feedback: In virtual fitness classes, instructors may not be able to provide personalized feedback to each individual, which may be a disadvantage for those who are new to a particular exercise.

Need for equipment: Some virtual fitness classes require users to have equipment, such as weights or a yoga mat, which can be an added expense for users.

Motivation: For some users, the lack of accountability and motivation that comes with attending an in-person class may be a disadvantage of virtual fitness classes. Users may find it difficult to stay motivated when working out alone at home.

Overall, virtual fitness classes are a convenient and flexible option for people with busy schedules or those who prefer to work out from home. However, users should be aware of the potential drawbacks and make sure they have a stable internet connection and any necessary equipment before attending a class.

Popular Classes

Virtual fitness classes have become increasingly popular over the years, especially in the wake of the COVID-19 pandemic, as people look for ways to stay active while staying at home. There are a wide variety of virtual fitness classes available, from yoga and pilates to high-intensity interval training (HIIT) and dance workouts. Here are some of the most popular classes:

Yoga: Yoga is a mind-body practice that involves physical poses, breathing techniques, and meditation. Virtual yoga classes are typically offered in a variety of styles, from gentle and restorative to more challenging vinyasa or power yoga classes. Some popular virtual yoga instructors include Adriene Mishler of Yoga With Adriene and Tara Stiles of Strala Yoga.

Pilates: Pilates is a low-impact form of exercise that focuses on building core strength, improving posture, and increasing flexibility. Virtual pilates classes often use props like resistance bands or small weights to enhance the workout. Popular virtual pilates instructors include Cassey Ho of Blogilates and Robin Long of The Balanced Life.

HIIT: High-intensity interval training (HIIT) is a type of workout that alternates short bursts of high-intensity exercise with periods of rest. Virtual HIIT classes are typically fast-paced and challenging, and can be done with little to no equipment. Some popular virtual HIIT instructors include Joe Wicks of The Body Coach and Kayla Itsines of Sweat.

Dance: Dance workouts are a fun and high-energy way to get your heart rate up and burn calories. Virtual dance classes range from ballet-inspired barre workouts to hip-hop and salsa classes. Some popular virtual dance instructors include Simone De La Rue of Body By Simone and Nicole Steen of POPSUGAR Fitness.

Bootcamp: Virtual bootcamp classes are designed to challenge your strength, endurance, and agility. They often use a combination of bodyweight exercises, resistance training, and cardio drills to provide a full-body workout. Popular virtual bootcamp instructors include Kaisa Keranen of KaisaFit and Charlee Atkins of Le Sweat.

Barre: Barre workouts combine ballet-inspired moves with strength and flexibility exercises. Virtual barre classes often use small props like hand weights or resistance bands to increase the intensity of the workout. Some popular virtual barre instructors include Mary Helen Bowers of Ballet Beautiful and Andrea Rogers of Xtend Barre.

Meditation: While not technically a fitness class, virtual meditation classes can be a great way to improve your mental and emotional well-being. Meditation can help reduce stress, anxiety, and depression, and improve focus and concentration. Popular virtual meditation instructors include Headspace and Calm.

These are just a few examples of the many virtual fitness classes available today. No matter what your fitness level or interests, there is likely a virtual class that will meet your needs and help you achieve your fitness goals.

Chapter 5: Pedometers
How They Work and What They Track

Pedometers are small devices that can be worn on the body to track the number of steps taken. They work by measuring the movement of the body and translating it into steps taken. Typically, pedometers are worn on the waistband, but they can also be clipped onto clothing or placed in a pocket.

The basic function of a pedometer is to track the number of steps taken. Some pedometers can also track distance traveled, calories burned, and other metrics related to physical activity. They do this by using an accelerometer, which is a sensor that measures movement.

When you take a step, the accelerometer detects the movement and counts it as a step. The pedometer then uses an algorithm to estimate the distance traveled based on the number of steps taken. The algorithm is based on the average stride length of the user, which is usually entered into the device manually.

Some pedometers also have additional features, such as the ability to track multiple activities, including cycling, swimming, and other forms of exercise. They may also have built-in memory to store data for several days or even weeks, allowing users to track their progress over time.

Pedometers can be simple or more advanced, with different features and tracking capabilities. Some pedometers have a digital display that shows the number of steps taken and other metrics, while others require syncing with a smartphone or computer to view data.

Overall, pedometers are a simple and easy-to-use tool for tracking physical activity. They can be a helpful tool for those looking to increase their activity level or monitor their progress towards fitness goals. However, they may not be as accurate as other tracking devices, and their functionality may be limited compared to more advanced tools.

Pros and Cons

Pedometers are simple and cost-effective tools to track the number of steps taken in a day. However, they also have their own set of advantages and disadvantages.

Pros:

Easy to use: Pedometers are easy to use and do not require any technical knowledge or complicated setup. Users simply need to attach them to their clothing, and they can start tracking their steps.

Inexpensive: Pedometers are relatively inexpensive and widely available. Users can purchase pedometers for as low as a few dollars, making them an affordable fitness tracking option.

Increased motivation: Seeing the number of steps taken in a day can increase motivation to be more active. This can be particularly helpful for people who are just starting their fitness journey or those who need a reminder to stay active throughout the day.

Track progress: Pedometers can help track progress over time. Users can set step goals and work towards achieving them, gradually increasing their daily step count.

Encourage physical activity: Pedometers can encourage people to be more physically active, which can have numerous health benefits, such as weight loss, improved cardiovascular health, and reduced risk of chronic diseases.

Cons:

Limited functionality: Pedometers only track the number of steps taken in a day and do not provide information on other metrics such as heart rate, calories burned, or distance traveled. Users who want a more comprehensive fitness tracking experience may need to use additional tools.

Inaccurate readings: Pedometers may not provide accurate readings for certain types of physical activity, such as cycling, swimming, or weightlifting. They may also be affected by factors such as user stride length, placement, or movement.

Lack of connectivity: Many pedometers do not offer connectivity options to smartphones or other devices. This means that users may need to manually track and input their data, which can be tedious.

Limited data analysis: Pedometers may not offer extensive data analysis or insights into user activity patterns or trends. This can make it difficult for users to identify areas for improvement or track progress over time.

Limited design options: Pedometers often have a limited range of designs and may not be suitable for all types of clothing or activities. Some users may find them uncomfortable or unappealing to wear.

Overall, pedometers can be a useful tool for people who want to track their steps and increase their physical activity. However, they do have their limitations, and users may need to supplement them with additional tools or devices to get a more comprehensive fitness tracking experience.

Popular Pedometers

In recent years, pedometers have become increasingly popular due to their ease of use and affordability. There are a variety of pedometer options available on the market, with different features and price points to suit different needs and budgets. In this section, we'll take a look at some of the most popular pedometers currently available.

Fitbit Inspire HR: The Fitbit Inspire HR is one of the most popular pedometers available today. It tracks steps, distance, calories burned, active minutes, and sleep, and can also monitor heart rate. The device syncs with the Fitbit app, which allows users to set goals and track progress over time. The Fitbit Inspire HR is also water-resistant and has a battery life of up to five days.

Garmin Vivofit 4: The Garmin Vivofit 4 is another popular pedometer option. It tracks steps, distance, calories burned, and sleep, and has a battery life of up to one year. The device syncs with the Garmin Connect app, which allows users to track progress and set goals.

Omron Alvita Ultimate Pedometer: The Omron Alvita Ultimate Pedometer is a popular choice for those who want a basic pedometer at an affordable price. It tracks steps, distance, and calories burned, and has a large, easy-to-read display. The device also includes a seven-day memory, which allows users to track progress over time.

3DFitBud Simple Step Counter: The 3DFitBud Simple Step Counter is a basic pedometer that tracks steps, distance, and calories burned. It has a compact design and can be easily attached to a waistband or pocket. The device has a battery life of up to 12 months and is affordably priced.

Xiaomi Mi Band 6: The Xiaomi Mi Band 6 is a popular pedometer option for those who want more advanced features at an affordable price. It tracks steps, distance, calories burned, heart rate, and sleep, and can also be used to monitor workouts. The device syncs with the Xiaomi Wear app, which allows users to set goals and track progress.

Overall, there are many popular pedometers available on the market today, with a range of features and price points to suit different needs and preferences. Whether you're looking for a basic pedometer or a more advanced device that can track heart rate and sleep, there is sure to be a pedometer out there that meets your needs.

Chapter 6: Exercise Video Games
How They Work and What They Offer

Exercise video games, also known as exergames, are a popular way to combine gaming and physical activity. They are designed to get players moving and provide an engaging and fun way to stay active. These games use motion controls and other sensors to track players' movements, making them feel like they are in the game.

Here is a closer look at how exercise video games work and what they offer:

Motion Controls

Most exercise video games use motion controls, which track players' movements using sensors or cameras. These controls allow players to interact with the game by mimicking real-world movements, such as swinging a tennis racket or doing a squat. The games use these movements to control characters, navigate environments, and perform actions.

Fitness Tracking

Many exercise video games come with built-in fitness tracking features. These features allow players to track their progress and set fitness goals. Players can track the number of calories they burn, the distance they travel, and the number of steps they take. They can also track their heart rate, which can help them stay within their target heart rate zone during exercise.

Game Modes

Exercise video games typically come with multiple game modes to keep players engaged. These modes can include solo play, multiplayer, and party modes. Solo play modes are designed for single players, while multiplayer modes allow players to compete against each other or work together to achieve a common goal. Party modes are designed for groups of people and provide a fun and social way to stay active.

Game Genres

Exercise video games come in a variety of genres, including sports, dance, and fitness. Sports games are designed to simulate real-world sports, such as tennis, golf, and basketball. Dance games are designed to get players moving to popular songs and teach them dance moves. Fitness games are designed to provide a full-body workout, with exercises such as yoga, cardio, and strength training.

Virtual Reality

Virtual reality (VR) is an emerging technology that is starting to make its way into exercise video games. VR provides an immersive experience that makes players feel like they are in the game. VR exercise video games typically require special equipment, such as a VR headset and hand controllers. The games use these devices to track players' movements and provide a fully immersive experience.

Accessibility

Exercise video games are generally accessible to people of all fitness levels and abilities. Most games offer multiple difficulty levels, making them suitable for beginners and more experienced players. Players can also modify the games to suit their fitness level, such as adjusting the intensity of the workouts.

Overall, exercise video games offer a fun and engaging way to stay active. They provide a variety of game modes, genres, and difficulty levels, making them accessible to people of all fitness levels and abilities. With built-in fitness tracking features, players can track their progress and stay motivated to achieve their fitness goals.

Pros and Cons

As with any form of exercise technology, exercise video games have their advantages and disadvantages. Here are some of the pros and cons of using exercise video games to get fit.

Pros:

Fun and engaging: One of the biggest advantages of exercise video games is that they are fun and engaging. They can help make exercise feel less like a chore and more like a game, which can be especially motivating for people who struggle to stay motivated to exercise.

Convenient: Exercise video games can be done at home, which can be especially convenient for people who don't have access to a gym or who don't have the time to go to a gym. They also don't require any special equipment, which can save money and space.

Suitable for all ages and fitness levels: Many exercise video games are suitable for all ages and fitness levels. They can be a great way for families to exercise together or for people who are just starting out on their fitness journey to get moving.

Variety: Exercise video games offer a wide variety of workouts, from dancing to yoga to strength training. This can help prevent boredom and keep things interesting.

Feedback: Many exercise video games offer feedback on performance, such as calories burned or steps taken. This can help people track their progress and stay motivated.

Cons:

Limited range of motion: Exercise video games often rely on a limited range of motion, which can be less effective than traditional forms of exercise that allow for a greater range of motion.

Limited resistance: Exercise video games also tend to have limited resistance, which can make them less effective at building strength and muscle mass.

Inaccurate tracking: Some exercise video games may not be accurate in tracking performance, which can make it difficult to measure progress and achieve fitness goals.

Sedentary gameplay: While exercise video games can be a great way to get moving, they still involve a significant amount of sedentary gameplay, which can be detrimental to health over the long term.

Cost: While exercise video games can be a cost-effective way to exercise at home, some games and equipment can be expensive, which can be a barrier for some people.

Overall, exercise video games can be a fun and convenient way to get moving, but they may not be the most effective form of exercise for everyone. It's important to consider your fitness goals and personal preferences when choosing a workout routine. Additionally, it's important to remember that exercise video games should not be the sole source of exercise but rather a complement to a well-rounded fitness program that includes aerobic exercise, strength training, and flexibility training.

Popular Games

Exercise video games have become increasingly popular in recent years as a fun and interactive way to stay active. From dancing games like Just Dance to sports games like Wii Sports, there are a variety of options to choose from. In this section, we'll explore some of the most popular exercise video games on the market.

Just Dance Just Dance is a popular dance game that allows players to follow along with on-screen dance moves set to popular music. The game is available on a variety of platforms, including the Nintendo Switch, PlayStation, and Xbox. Players can select from a variety of songs and difficulty levels, making it a great option for all skill levels.

Wii Sports Wii Sports is a classic exercise game that was first released in 2006 for the Nintendo Wii. The game features a variety of sports, including boxing, tennis, and bowling, that require players to move their bodies to play. The game is known for its motion-based controls, which allow players to swing a virtual tennis racket or throw a virtual bowling ball using their actual movements.

Ring Fit Adventure Ring Fit Adventure is a newer exercise game that was released in 2019 for the Nintendo Switch. The game comes with a special controller called the Ring-Con, which players use to complete exercises like squats, presses, and pulls. The game features a variety of levels and boss battles, making it a fun and challenging way to stay active.

Zumba Fitness Zumba Fitness is a dance game that's based on the popular Zumba exercise program. The game features a variety of dance routines set to Latin and international music, and players can select from a variety of modes and difficulty levels. The game is available on a variety of platforms, including the Wii, Xbox, and PlayStation.

Beat Saber Beat Saber is a newer exercise game that was released in 2018 for virtual reality platforms like the Oculus Quest and PlayStation VR. The game requires players to slash through oncoming obstacles with virtual lightsabers, providing a fun and fast-paced workout. The game features a variety of levels and difficulty modes, making it a great option for players of all skill levels.

Overall, exercise video games provide a fun and engaging way to stay active. With a variety of options to choose from, there's a game out there for everyone. Whether you're a fan of dancing, sports, or virtual reality, there's an exercise game that will help you stay fit and have fun at the same time.

Chapter 7: Smart Watches
How They Work and What They Track

Smartwatches have become increasingly popular in recent years due to their many features and functionalities. One of their most important features is their ability to track various aspects of physical activity, making them a valuable tool for fitness enthusiasts and health-conscious individuals alike. In this section, we will explore how smartwatches work and what they track.

Smartwatches are essentially miniature computers that can be worn on the wrist. They have a range of sensors and features that allow them to track various aspects of physical activity, such as steps taken, distance traveled, and calories burned. Some models are also equipped with heart rate monitors, which provide continuous or periodic heart rate measurements throughout the day. This data can be used to monitor heart rate trends, which can be helpful for identifying potential health issues or assessing overall fitness levels.

In addition to tracking physical activity, smartwatches can also track other health metrics, such as sleep quality and duration, stress levels, and even blood oxygen levels. Some models are also equipped with GPS functionality, which can be used to track outdoor activities such as running or cycling.

One of the most valuable aspects of smartwatches is their ability to sync with various apps and services. Many popular fitness apps, such as Fitbit and Strava, have smartwatch compatibility, allowing users to easily track their workouts and monitor their progress. Some smartwatches also offer built-in coaching and training features, which can provide users with personalized workout plans and guidance.

Overall, smartwatches are a versatile tool for tracking physical activity and monitoring various health metrics. They are easy to use and offer a wide range of features, making them an excellent choice for anyone looking to stay active and maintain a healthy lifestyle.

Pros and Cons

Smart watches are becoming increasingly popular as a fitness tracking device due to their versatility and convenience. However, there are both advantages and disadvantages to using them for fitness tracking.

Pros:

Convenience: Smart watches are a convenient way to track your fitness activities since they are always on your wrist. This makes them an excellent option for those who do not want to carry their phone around while exercising.

Versatility: Smart watches offer a wide range of fitness tracking features. They can track steps, distance, calories burned, heart rate, and other activities like swimming, cycling, and even sleep.

Goal Setting: Many smart watches allow you to set fitness goals and track your progress. This can be a great motivator to help you stay on track with your fitness journey.

Integration: Smart watches can be integrated with other fitness apps and devices, making it easy to track your fitness activities across different platforms.

Cons:

Price: Smart watches can be expensive, and not everyone can afford to invest in one just for fitness tracking.

Battery Life: Some smart watches have limited battery life, which can be an issue if you are tracking multiple activities throughout the day.

Accuracy: While smart watches are generally accurate, they may not be as precise as other devices like chest straps or other dedicated fitness trackers.

Data Overload: With so much data available, it can be overwhelming to track and interpret the information, which may not be suitable for everyone.

Reliance on Technology: Smart watches are dependent on technology, and if they fail, it can be challenging to track your fitness activities.

Overall, smart watches are an excellent option for those who want a versatile and convenient way to track their fitness activities. However, they may not be the best option for everyone due to their cost, battery life, and accuracy limitations. It is essential to consider your fitness goals and preferences before investing in a smart watch.

Popular Watches

As smartwatches have become increasingly popular in recent years, there are many options to choose from. Here are some of the most popular smartwatches on the market:

Apple Watch The Apple Watch is one of the most popular smartwatches available. It offers a range of health and fitness features, such as heart rate monitoring, step tracking, and workout tracking. It also offers an ECG feature that can help detect irregular heart rhythms. The Apple Watch is compatible with the iPhone and has a range of apps, including fitness and workout apps.

Samsung Galaxy Watch The Samsung Galaxy Watch is another popular option. It has a wide range of health and fitness features, such as heart rate monitoring, sleep tracking, and stress tracking. It also offers automatic workout detection and can track over 40 different exercises. The Samsung Galaxy Watch is compatible with both Android and iOS devices and has a range of apps, including fitness and workout apps.

Fitbit Versa The Fitbit Versa is a popular fitness-focused smartwatch. It offers a range of health and fitness features, such as heart rate monitoring, step tracking, and workout tracking. It also offers personalized on-screen coaching and can track over 15 different exercises. The Fitbit

Versa is compatible with both Android and iOS devices and has a range of fitness and workout apps.

Garmin Forerunner The Garmin Forerunner is a popular option for runners and other athletes. It offers a range of health and fitness features, such as heart rate monitoring, GPS tracking, and workout tracking. It also offers personalized coaching and can track over 20 different exercises. The Garmin Forerunner is compatible with both Android and iOS devices and has a range of fitness and workout apps.

Fossil Gen 5 The Fossil Gen 5 is a popular smartwatch that offers a range of health and fitness features, such as heart rate monitoring and step tracking. It also offers workout tracking and can track over 20 different exercises. The Fossil Gen 5 is compatible with both Android and iOS devices and has a range of apps, including fitness and workout apps.

Huawei Watch GT 2 The Huawei Watch GT 2 is a popular smartwatch that offers a range of health and fitness features, such as heart rate monitoring, sleep tracking, and stress tracking. It also offers workout tracking and can track over 15 different exercises. The Huawei Watch GT 2 is compatible with both Android and iOS devices and has a range of apps, including fitness and workout apps.

TicWatch Pro 3 The TicWatch Pro 3 is a popular smartwatch that offers a range of health and fitness features, such as heart rate monitoring and sleep tracking. It also offers workout tracking and can track over 10 different exercises. The TicWatch Pro 3 is compatible with both Android and iOS devices and has a range of apps, including fitness and workout apps.

Withings Steel HR The Withings Steel HR is a popular hybrid smartwatch that offers a range of health and fitness features, such as heart rate monitoring, step tracking, and workout tracking. It also offers sleep tracking and has a long battery life. The Withings Steel HR is compatible with both Android and iOS devices and has a range of fitness and workout apps.

Amazfit Bip S The Amazfit Bip S is a popular budget-friendly smartwatch that offers a range of health and fitness features, such as heart rate monitoring and step tracking. It also offers workout tracking and can track over 10 different exercises. The Amazfit Bip S is compatible with both Android and iOS devices and has a range of apps, including fitness and workout apps.

Honor Band 6 The Honor Band 6 is a fitness tracker that offers a range of features, including heart rate monitoring, sleep tracking, and workout tracking. The device has a 1.47-inch AMOLED display that is crisp and easy to read. It also has a long battery life, with up to 14 days of use on a single charge. The Honor Band 6 can be paired with the Huawei Health app, which allows users to track their progress and set fitness goals.

Garmin Venu The Garmin Venu is a smartwatch that offers a range of fitness features, including GPS tracking, heart rate monitoring, and workout tracking. The device also has a number of smartwatch features, such as notifications and music control. The Venu has a vibrant AMOLED display that is easy to read, and the battery can last up to five days on a single charge. The watch can be paired with the Garmin Connect app, which provides a range of insights and suggestions based on the user's activity.

Samsung Galaxy Watch Active 2 The Samsung Galaxy Watch Active 2 is a smartwatch that offers a range of fitness features, including GPS tracking, heart rate monitoring, and workout tracking. The device also has a number of smartwatch features, such as notifications and music control. The watch has a sleek design and a bright, clear display. The battery can last up to two days on a single charge. The watch can be paired with the Samsung Health app, which allows users to track their progress and set fitness goals.

Fitbit Charge 4 The Fitbit Charge 4 is a fitness tracker that offers a range of features, including GPS tracking, heart rate monitoring, and workout tracking. The device also has a number of smartwatch features, such as notifications and music control. The Charge 4 has a bright OLED display that is easy to read, and the battery can last up to seven days on a single charge. The device can be paired with the Fitbit app, which provides a range of insights and suggestions based on the user's activity.

Polar Vantage V2 The Polar Vantage V2 is a smartwatch that offers a range of fitness features, including GPS tracking, heart rate monitoring, and workout tracking. The device also has a number of smartwatch features, such as notifications and music control. The watch has a clear, easy-to-read display and a long battery life, with up to 40 hours of use in training mode. The watch can be paired with the Polar Flow app, which provides a range of insights and suggestions based on the user's activity.

Suunto 7 The Suunto 7 is a smartwatch that offers a range of fitness features, including GPS tracking, heart rate monitoring, and workout tracking. The device also has a number of smartwatch features, such as notifications and music control. The Suunto 7 has a bright, clear display and a long battery life, with up to two days of use on a single charge. The watch can be paired with the Suunto app, which provides a range of insights and suggestions based on the user's activity.

Overall, there are many smartwatches on the market that offer a range of features for fitness enthusiasts. When choosing a smartwatch, it's important to consider the specific features that are most important to you, as well as the overall design and battery life of the device. By doing so, you can find a smartwatch that fits your needs and helps you stay on track with your fitness goals.

Chapter 8: Comparing and Contrasting Methods
Summary of Pros and Cons

In this chapter, we have examined a variety of fitness technologies, each with its own unique advantages and disadvantages. In this section, we will summarize the key pros and cons of each technology to help you make an informed decision about which technology might be best for your fitness goals.

Fitness Trackers: Pros:

Provides accurate measurement of physical activity levels throughout the day.

Can track various fitness metrics like steps, calories burned, heart rate, sleep, etc.

Can help motivate individuals to move more and be active.

Often have long battery life and durable design for long-term use.

Cons:

Some trackers may not be as accurate as others.

Limited ability to track specific exercises and activities.

May be uncomfortable to wear for long periods of time.

Can be expensive, especially for high-end models.

Exercise Apps: Pros:

Offer a wide variety of exercises and workouts to suit all fitness levels.

Can be easily customized to meet individual fitness goals.

Provide guidance and motivation through in-app features and social communities.

Can be easily accessed and used at home or on-the-go.

Cons:

Require a reliable internet connection.

Some apps may require a subscription or in-app purchases for access to all features.

May not provide personalized coaching or form correction.

Can be distracting or difficult to follow for beginners.

Smart Home Gym Equipment: Pros:

Provides the convenience of a gym at home.

Offers a variety of exercises and workouts in a single machine.

Often provides personalized coaching and form correction.

Can track progress and adjust workouts accordingly.

Cons:

Expensive initial investment for high-end models.

May take up a significant amount of space.

Limited ability to perform some exercises compared to traditional gym equipment.

May require professional installation or technical support.

Virtual Fitness Classes: Pros:

Offer a wide variety of classes to suit all fitness levels and interests.

Can be accessed from anywhere with an internet connection.

Provide motivation through live instructors and virtual communities.

Can be more affordable than traditional gym memberships.

Cons:

May require additional equipment or space to participate.

May not provide personalized coaching or form correction.

Require a reliable internet connection.

May not provide the same sense of community or camaraderie as traditional gym classes.

Pedometers: Pros:

Provides an easy way to track daily physical activity levels.

Often simple and affordable.

Can motivate individuals to move more throughout the day.

Can provide helpful data for fitness goal setting.

Cons:

May not be as accurate as other fitness technologies.

Limited ability to track specific exercises and activities.

May not provide real-time feedback or motivation during physical activity.

May not provide additional features beyond step tracking.

Exercise Video Games: Pros:

Offers a fun and interactive way to exercise.

Can be accessed from home.

Often provides a sense of accomplishment and progression.

Can offer a wide variety of activities and fitness games.

Cons:

May require additional equipment or space to play.

May not provide the same level of physical activity as traditional exercise.

May not provide personalized coaching or form correction.

May be distracting or difficult to follow for beginners.

Smart Watches: Pros:

Provides a variety of fitness tracking features.

Often includes other helpful features like GPS and mobile payment options.

Stylish and can be worn in a variety of settings.

Can be a great tool for tracking overall health and wellness.

Cons:

May be expensive, especially for high-end models.

May not provide the same level of accuracy as dedicated fitness trackers.

Limited ability to track specific exercises and activities.

May require frequent charging or maintenance.

In summary, each method of tracking fitness has its own set of pros and cons. Fitness trackers offer convenience and accuracy, but they can be costly and may not provide a complete picture of overall health. Exercise apps offer a wide range of features and customization options, but they require consistent smartphone usage and can be distracting during workouts. Smart home gym equipment provides a personalized workout experience and saves space, but can be expensive and may not offer the same level of motivation as group fitness classes. Virtual fitness classes offer the benefits of group fitness in the comfort of home, but may not provide personalized feedback and require a stable internet connection. Pedometers are affordable and offer simple tracking, but may not be as accurate as other methods and do not provide detailed workout feedback. Exercise video games offer an immersive and fun workout experience, but may not provide as much physical activity as other methods and require the purchase of additional equipment. Smart watches provide a comprehensive view of fitness and health, but can be expensive and may require regular charging.

  When choosing a method of tracking fitness, it is important to consider personal goals, preferences, and budget. Some individuals may prefer the convenience of a fitness tracker or the personalized workout experience of smart home gym equipment, while others may prefer the social aspect of virtual fitness classes or the fun of exercise video games. Pedometers and smart watches may be better suited for those looking for simple and comprehensive tracking, respectively. It is important to evaluate the pros and cons of each method and choose one that fits individual needs and preferences.

Criteria for Comparison

When it comes to choosing the best exercise method for you, there are several criteria to consider. These criteria are useful in comparing and contrasting the different exercise methods available and determining which method is the best fit for your needs and goals. Here are some of the most important criteria to consider:

Accessibility: One of the most important criteria to consider is accessibility. How easy is it to access and use the exercise method? Does it require expensive equipment, specialized training, or a specific location? Are the exercises difficult to learn or perform? The more accessible an exercise method is, the more likely you are to stick with it long-term.

Effectiveness: Another important criteria is effectiveness. How effective is the exercise method at achieving your goals? Does it provide a full-body workout or focus on specific muscle groups? Does it help you build strength, flexibility, or cardiovascular endurance? Consider your goals and choose an exercise method that will help you achieve them.

Fun and enjoyment: An often overlooked criteria is how much fun and enjoyment the exercise method provides. If you enjoy the exercises, you're more likely to stick with the routine long-term. Consider whether the exercise method is enjoyable and whether you look forward to doing it regularly.

Cost: Cost is another important criteria to consider. Some exercise methods, such as gym memberships or personal trainers, can be expensive. Other methods, such as exercise apps, may be more affordable or even free. Consider your budget and choose an exercise method that is affordable and fits your financial situation.

Variety: Variety is also important when it comes to exercise. Doing the same exercises day in and day out can quickly become boring and may lead to a lack of motivation. Look for exercise methods that offer a variety of exercises and workouts to keep you engaged and motivated.

Personalization: Finally, consider whether the exercise method can be personalized to meet your specific needs and goals. Can you modify the workouts to meet your fitness level or accommodate any injuries or limitations you may have? The more personalized the exercise method is, the more likely you are to stick with it and see results.

By considering these criteria, you can better compare and contrast the different exercise methods available and choose the one that is the best fit for your needs and goals. Remember, the best exercise method is the one you enjoy and will stick with long-term.

Recommendations for Different Needs

When it comes to selecting a fitness method, there are several factors to consider, such as personal goals, fitness level, schedule, and budget. Here are some recommendations for different needs:

Busy Schedules: If you have a busy schedule and find it challenging to make time for workouts, then high-intensity interval training (HIIT) or virtual fitness classes might be the best option for you. HIIT workouts are short, but they can be very effective, and you can do them anywhere, even at home. Virtual fitness classes offer flexibility, and you can participate in them from anywhere, at any time, as long as you have an internet connection.

Low-Impact Workouts: If you are recovering from an injury or looking for a low-impact workout, then pedometers, smartwatches, or exercise bikes might be a good option for you. Pedometers and smartwatches track your steps and heart rate and can help you monitor your progress. Exercise bikes offer a low-impact workout that is gentle on the joints.

Strength Training: If you want to build muscle and get stronger, then home gym equipment or exercise apps might be the best option for you. Home gym equipment offers a wide range of strength-training options, from resistance bands to weight machines, while exercise apps provide customizable workouts that target specific muscle groups.

Interactive Workouts: If you enjoy interactive and immersive workouts, then exercise video games might be the best option for you. Exercise video games offer a fun and engaging way to work out, and they can be a great way to motivate yourself to exercise.

Budget-Conscious: If you're on a tight budget, then pedometers or exercise apps might be the best option for you. Pedometers are relatively inexpensive and can help you monitor your steps and progress. Exercise apps offer customizable workouts at a fraction of the cost of gym memberships or personal trainers.

Overall, there is no one-size-fits-all approach to fitness, and the best option for you will depend on your personal goals, fitness level, schedule, and budget. It's essential to choose a method that you enjoy and can stick with over the long term. By considering your needs and preferences, you can find the perfect fitness method to help you achieve your goals.

Conclusion

Recap of Importance of Physical Activity

Throughout this guide, we have explored various methods of incorporating physical activity into our lives, including exercise apps, smart home gym equipment, virtual fitness classes, pedometers, exercise video games, and smart watches. While each method has its own pros and cons, they all share a common goal: to encourage and facilitate physical activity.

Regular physical activity is crucial for maintaining good health and preventing chronic diseases such as heart disease, stroke, diabetes, and certain cancers. It can also help manage mental health conditions like anxiety and depression, boost energy levels, and improve overall quality of life.

However, despite the many benefits of physical activity, many people struggle to find the time or motivation to exercise. That is where these various methods come in. By providing convenience, variety, and interactive features, they make it easier and more enjoyable to incorporate physical activity into our daily lives.

But while these methods can certainly be helpful, it is important to keep in mind that they are not a replacement for a well-rounded, balanced approach to physical activity.

Incorporating other types of activity, such as outdoor activities or group sports, can provide additional health benefits and social connections.

It is also important to remember that physical activity is just one part of a healthy lifestyle. Proper nutrition, stress management, and sufficient sleep are also crucial for overall health and wellbeing.

In conclusion, this guide has provided a comprehensive overview of various methods for incorporating physical activity into our lives. By understanding the pros and cons of each method and considering our own personal needs and preferences, we can make informed choices about how to stay active and healthy. But no matter which methods we choose, the most important thing is that we prioritize and prioritize regular physical activity as an essential component of our daily lives.

Final Thoughts and Recommendations

Physical activity is essential for leading a healthy and fulfilling life. However, with our busy schedules and sedentary lifestyles, finding the time and motivation to exercise can be a challenge. Fortunately, technology has made it easier than ever to incorporate physical activity into our daily routines. From smart home gym equipment to virtual fitness classes, pedometers to exercise video games, and smartwatches to activity trackers, there are a variety of tools available to help us achieve our fitness goals.

As we have seen in this guide, each method of incorporating physical activity into our lives has its own unique set of advantages and disadvantages. Some methods may be better suited for certain individuals, depending on their preferences, fitness goals, and lifestyles. It is important to carefully evaluate each option and consider the pros and cons before deciding on a particular method.

Regardless of the method, it is important to stay motivated and committed to achieving your fitness goals. Setting achievable goals, tracking progress, and celebrating milestones along the way can help you stay motivated and focused. Additionally, finding an accountability partner or joining a community of like-minded individuals can provide the necessary support and encouragement to stay on track.

In conclusion, incorporating physical activity into our daily routines is essential for leading a healthy and fulfilling life. Technology has made it easier than ever to stay active, with a wide range of tools and resources available to help us achieve our fitness goals. By carefully evaluating the pros and cons of each method, setting achievable goals, and staying motivated and committed, we can all achieve a healthier and more active lifestyle.

THE END

Potential References

Introduction:

World Health Organization. (2018). Physical activity. Retrieved from https://www.who.int/news-room/fact-sheets/detail/physical-activity

Centers for Disease Control and Prevention. (2020). How much physical activity do adults need? Retrieved from https://www.cdc.gov/physicalactivity/basics/adults/index.htm

Chapter 1: Fitness Trackers:

International Data Corporation. (2020). Worldwide wearables market to nearly double by 2024, according to IDC. Retrieved from https://www.idc.com/getdoc.jsp?containerId=prUS46762220

American Council on Exercise. (2019). Are fitness trackers accurate? Retrieved from https://www.acefitness.org/education-and-resources/lifestyle/blog/7385/are-fitness-trackers-accurate/

Pevnick, J. M., & Jasuja, G. K. (2018). The growing role of wearables in managing chronic disease. Mhealth, 4, 1-14.

Chapter 2: Exercise Apps:

Statista. (2020). Number of health and fitness apps available in the Apple App Store from 1st quarter 2015 to 3rd quarter

2020. Retrieved from https://www.statista.com/statistics/779910/health-fitness-apps-available-ios-worldwide/

Liu, L., Miguel Cruz, A., Rios Rincon, A., Buttar, V., Ranson, Q., Goertzen, D., ... & Jadad, A. R. (2017). What factors determine therapists' acceptance of new technologies for rehabilitation—a study using the Unified Theory of Acceptance and Use of Technology (UTAUT). Disability and rehabilitation, 39(20), 2041-2048.

Fanning, J., Mullen, S. P., McAuley, E., & Rhodes, R. E. (2012). Increasing physical activity with mobile devices: a meta-analysis. Journal of medical Internet research, 14(6), e161.

Chapter 3: Smart Home Gym Equipment:

Grand View Research. (2020). Smart home gym equipment market size worth $7.01 billion by 2027. Retrieved from https://www.grandviewresearch.com/press-release/global-smart-home-gym-equipment-market

Vartanian, O., & Santanam, R. (2020). Innovative uses of smart technology in the home fitness industry. Journal of Consumer Marketing, 37(7), 858-870.

American College of Sports Medicine. (2018). Selecting and effectively using home exercise equipment. Retrieved from https://www.acsm.org/docs/default-source/files-for-resource-library/selecting-and-effectively-using-home-exercise-equipment.pdf?sfvrsn=4c417f7b_2

Chapter 4: Virtual Fitness Classes:

Market Research Future. (2018). Virtual fitness market research report—global forecast till 2023. Retrieved from https://www.marketresearchfuture.com/reports/virtual-fitness-market-6888

American Council on Exercise. (2020). Are virtual workouts effective? Retrieved from https://www.acefitness.org/education-and-resources/professional/expert-articles/7513/are-virtual-workouts-effective/

The New York Times. (2020). The best virtual and online fitness classes for staying fit during the pandemic. Retrieved from https://www.nytimes.com/wirecutter/reviews/best-virtual-and-online-fitness-classes/

Chapter 5: Pedometers

Tudor-Locke, C., & Lutes, L. (2009). Why do pedometers work?: A reflection upon the factors related to successfully increasing physical activity. Sports Medicine, 39(12), 981-993. https://doi.org/10.2165/11319600-000000000-00000

Kang, M., Marshall, S. J., & Barreira, T. V. (2009). Effect of pedometer-based physical activity interventions: A meta-analysis. Research Quarterly for Exercise and Sport, 80(3),

648-655. https://doi.org/10.1080/02701367.2009.10599609

Chapter 6: Exercise Video Games

Lyons, E. J., Tate, D. F., & Ward, D. S. (2012). Energy expenditure and enjoyment of common children's exergames. Games for Health Journal, 1(3), 205-210. https://doi.org/10.1089/g4h.2012.0014

Peng, W., Crouse, J., & Lin, J.-H. (2013). Using active video games for physical activity promotion: A systematic review of the current state of research. Health Education & Behavior, 40(2), 171-192. https://doi.org/10.1177/1090198112455777

Chapter 7: Smart Watches

Shcherbina, A., Mattsson, C. M., Waggott, D., Salisbury, H., Christle, J. W., Hastie, T., ... & Ashley, E. A. (2017). Accuracy in wrist-worn, sensor-based measurements of heart rate and energy expenditure in a diverse cohort. Journal of Personalized Medicine, 7(2), 3. https://doi.org/10.3390/jpm7020003

Montes, J., Young, L. R., & Leckie, R. L. (2019). Assessing the validity of wearable fitness trackers' measurement of sleep and sleep stages: A systematic review and meta-analysis. Sleep Medicine Reviews, 45, 68-82. https://doi.org/10.1016/j.smrv.2019.02.001

Chapter 8: Comparing and Contrasting Methods

Bassett Jr, D. R., Toth, L. P., LaMunion, S. R., & Crouter, S. E. (2017). Step counting: A review of measurement considerations and health-related applications. Sports Medicine, 47(7), 1303-1315. https://doi.org/10.1007/s40279-016-0663-8

Rosenberger, M. E., Buman, M. P., Haskell, W. L., McConnell, M. V., & Carstensen, L. L. (2016). Twenty-four hours of sleep, sedentary behavior, and physical activity with nine wearable devices. Medicine & Science in Sports & Exercise, 48(3), 457-465. https://doi.org/10.1249/MSS.0000000000000778

Conclusion

Physical Activity Guidelines Advisory Committee. (2018). 2018 Physical Activity Guidelines Advisory Committee Scientific Report. US Department of Health and Human Services. https://health.gov/sites/default/files/2019-09/PAG_Advisory_Committee_Report.pdf

Centers for Disease Control and Prevention. (2015). Physical Activity and Health. https://www.cdc.gov/healthyschools/physicalactivity/index.htm

www.ingramcontent.com/pod-product-compliance
Lightning Source LLC
LaVergne TN
LVHW010411070526
838199LV00065B/5947